20 FUN FACTS ABOUT THE MUSCULAR SYSTEM

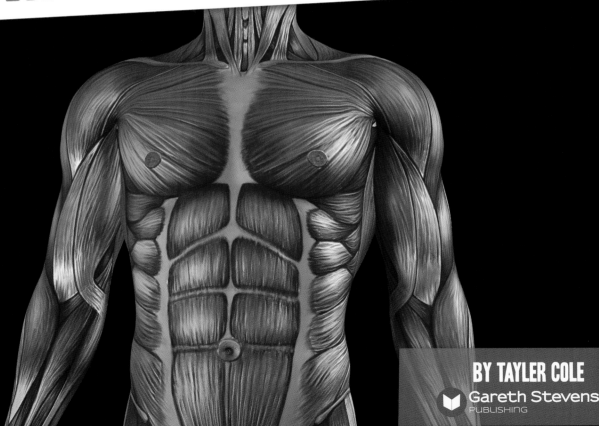

BY TAYLER COLE

Gareth Stevens
PUBLISHING

Please visit our website, www.garethstevens.com. For a free color catalog of all our high-quality books, call toll free 1-800-542-2595 or fax 1-877-542-2596.

Library of Congress Cataloging-in-Publication Data

Names: Cole, Tayler, author.
Title: 20 fun facts about the muscular system / Tayler Cole.
Other titles: Twenty fun facts about the muscular system
Description: New York : Gareth Stevens Publishing, [2019] | Series: Fun fact
   file: body systems | Includes bibliographical references and index.
Identifiers: LCCN 2018026464| ISBN 9781538229231 (library bound) | ISBN
   9781538232767 (pbk.) | ISBN 9781538232774 (6 pack)
Subjects: LCSH: Muscles–Juvenile literature.
Classification: LCC QM151 .C65 2019 | DDC 612.7/4–dc23
LC record available at https://lccn.loc.gov/2018026464

First Edition

Published in 2019 by
Gareth Stevens Publishing
111 East 14th Street, Suite 349
New York, NY 10003

Designer: Sarah Liddell
Editor: Meta Manchester

Photo credits: Cover, pp. 1 (main), 18, 22 Sebastian Kaulitzki/Shutterstock.com; file folder used throughout David Smart/Shutterstock.com; binder clip used throughout luckyraccoon/Shutterstock.com; wood grain background used throughout ARENA Creative/Shutterstock.com; p. 5 Sakurra/Shutterstock.com; p. 6 (main) adike/Shutterstock.com; pp. 6 (inset), 8 (inset) Choksawatdikorn/Shutterstock.com; p. 7 stihii/Shutterstock.com; pp. 8 (main), 11 sciencepics/Shutterstock.com; p. 9 (main) Liya Graphics/Shutterstock.com; p. 9 (inset) De Agostini Picture Library/Contributor/De Agostini/Getty Images; p. 10 Nerthuz/Shutterstock.com; p. 12 joshya/Shutterstock.com; p. 13 Africa Studio/Shutterstock.com; p. 14 Jacek Chabraszewski/Shutterstock.com; p. 15 fotogestoeber/Shutterstock.com; p. 16 Alila Medical Media/Shutterstock.com; p. 17 Nataly Mayak/Shutterstock.com; p. 19 Katya Shut/Shutterstock.com; p. 20 Voyagerix/Shutterstock.com; p. 21 SVETLANA VERBINSKAYA/Shutterstock.com; p. 23 decade3d - anatomy online/Shutterstock.com; p. 24 Rob Marmion/Shutterstock.com; p. 25 wavebreakmedia/Shutterstock.com; p. 26 Fer Gregory/Shutterstock.com; p. 27 NASA/Discostu/Wikimedia Commons; p. 29 Sergey Novikov/Shutterstock.com.

Printed in the United States of America

CPSIA compliance information: Batch #CW19GS: For further information contact Gareth Stevens, New York, New York at 1-800-542-2595.

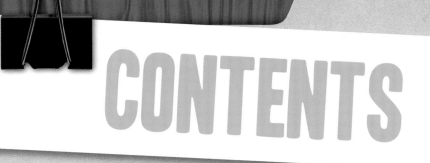

CONTENTS

Words in the glossary appear in **bold** type the first time they are used in the text.

SO MANY MUSCLES!

When most people think of the muscular system, they usually think of skeletal muscles. These are the muscles that make your body move. Skeletal muscles are attached to your bones by **tendons**, usually on either side of a **joint**.

Your body has other types of muscle, too! Some of your **organs** are made of smooth muscle, and your heart is made mostly of **cardiac** muscle. Each type of muscle has a different job in the body. Are you ready to learn more about muscles?

TYPES OF MUSCLE TISSUE

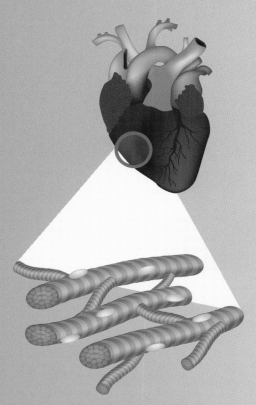

CARDIAC MUSCLE

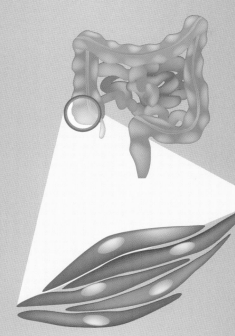

SMOOTH MUSCLE

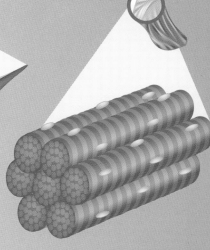

SKELETAL MUSCLE

Muscles make your body move by contracting, or getting shorter, and relaxing, or getting longer.

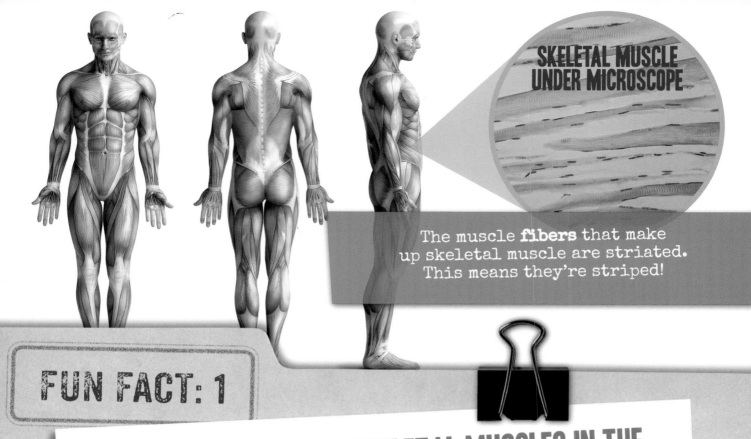

The muscle **fibers** that make up skeletal muscle are striated. This means they're striped!

FUN FACT: 1

THERE ARE ABOUT 650 SKELETAL MUSCLES IN THE HUMAN BODY!

There's no exact number because scientists can't agree on which muscles are a single muscle and which are more than one muscle. It's also been found that some people have more muscles than others!

MUSCLE MOVEMENT

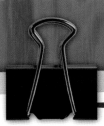

YOUR SKELETAL MUSCLES ARE UNDER YOUR CONTROL!

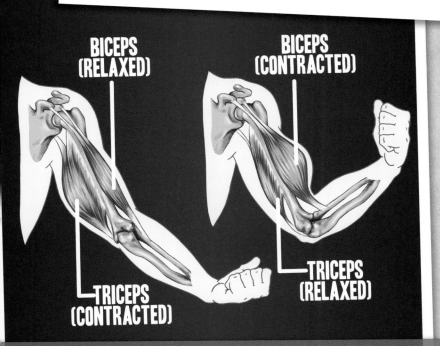

BICEPS
(RELAXED)

BICEPS
(CONTRACTED)

TRICEPS
(CONTRACTED)

TRICEPS
(RELAXED)

Skeletal muscles work in pairs. To bend your arm at your elbow, your brain tells your biceps to contract and your triceps to relax. To straighten your arm, your triceps contract while your biceps relax.

Skeletal muscles are also called voluntary muscles. Voluntary means you can decide to do or not do something. If you want to move your body, your brain will send a message to your skeletal muscles.

YOU CAN'T CONTROL YOUR SMOOTH MUSCLES, EVEN IF YOU TRY!

These muscles are also called involuntary muscles. They do what your brain and body tell them to do without you needing to think about it. As smooth muscles contract and relax, they push blood or food through your system!

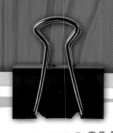

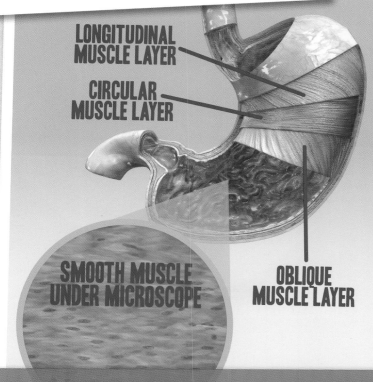

LONGITUDINAL MUSCLE LAYER

CIRCULAR MUSCLE LAYER

SMOOTH MUSCLE UNDER MICROSCOPE

OBLIQUE MUSCLE LAYER

Smooth muscles are found inside hollow organs, such as your stomach, and also line your **intestines** and most blood **vessels**. They're usually found in layers.

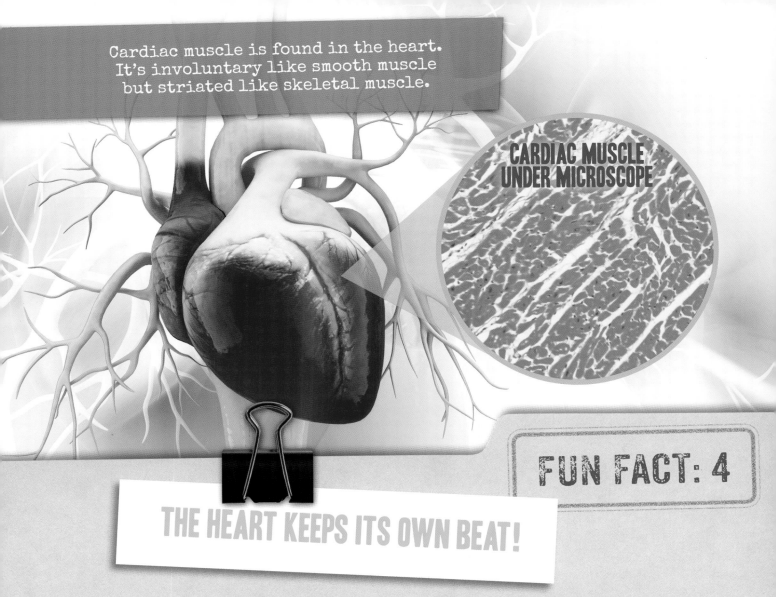

Cardiac muscle is found in the heart. It's involuntary like smooth muscle but striated like skeletal muscle.

CARDIAC MUSCLE UNDER MICROSCOPE

FUN FACT: 4

THE HEART KEEPS ITS OWN BEAT!

The heart is an involuntary muscle, so you don't need to think about making it beat. An electrical **impulse** in the muscle tells it to contract and relax. This is what makes the heart beat!

9

THE LEFT SIDE OF YOUR BRAIN CONTROLS THE MUSCLES ON THE RIGHT SIDE OF YOUR BODY!

Similarly, the right side of your brain controls the muscles on the left side of your body! This is because of something called crossed control.

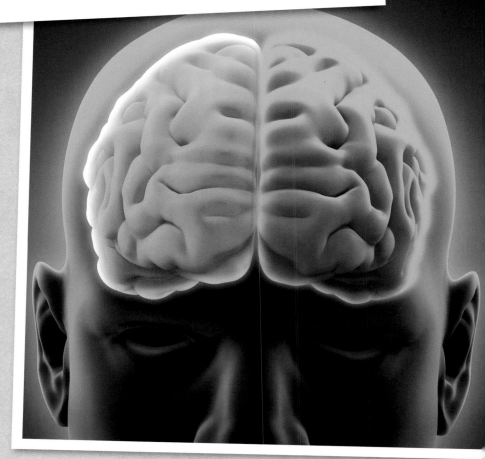

MESSAGES FROM THE BRAIN

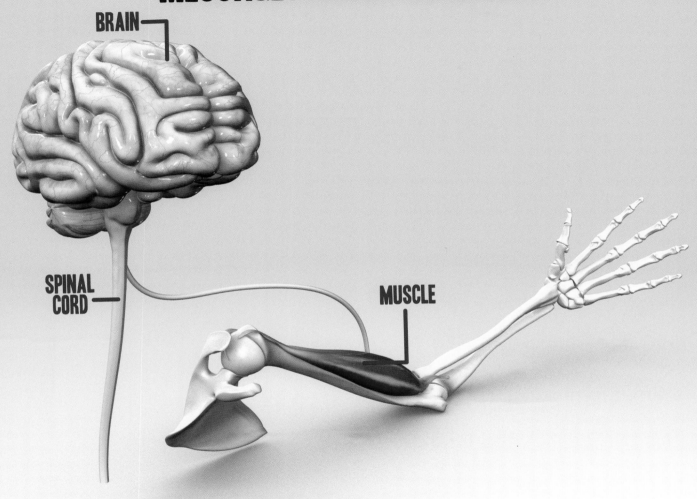

BRAIN

SPINAL CORD

MUSCLE

The brain sends messages to the muscles through the spinal cord and other parts of the nervous system. More messages are sent for more complicated movements.

GROSS MOTION

FOOD MAKES YOUR MUSCLES MOVE!

The walls of your throat, stomach, and intestines are made of smooth muscle. When food rubs against them, the muscles contract. This pushes the food through the digestive system. These muscles movements are called peristalsis.

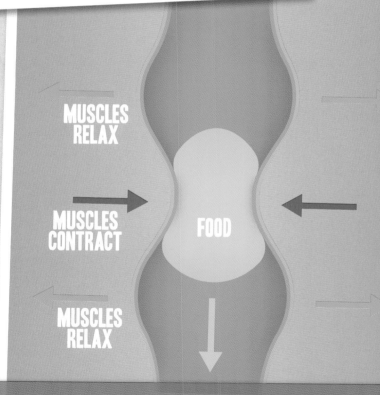

MUSCLES RELAX

MUSCLES CONTRACT

FOOD

MUSCLES RELAX

A contraction must be followed by relaxation so food has room to move.

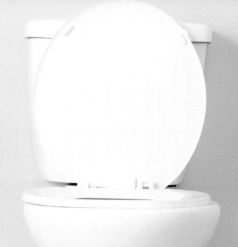

Most children are ready to begin potty training when they're around 2 years old.

MUSCLES LET YOU KNOW IF YOU HAVE TO GO!

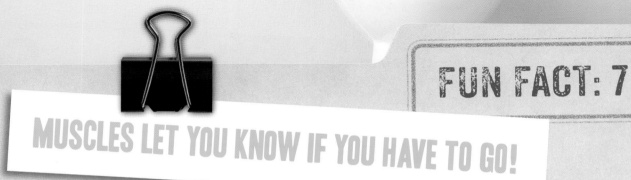

The bladder is lined with involuntary smooth muscle. When it's full, these muscles contract and the inner **sphincter** in the bladder relaxes, making you feel like you have to go. When you go to the bathroom, the outer sphincter relaxes to release urine. The outer sphincter is a voluntary muscle that you learn to control when potty training!

13

TURN UP THE HEAT!

FUN FACT: 8

YOUR MUSCLES ARE YOUR BODY'S HEATER!

Muscles get energy by breaking down special **nutrients**. This process creates heat. When you exercise, the process happens much faster and more heat is created.

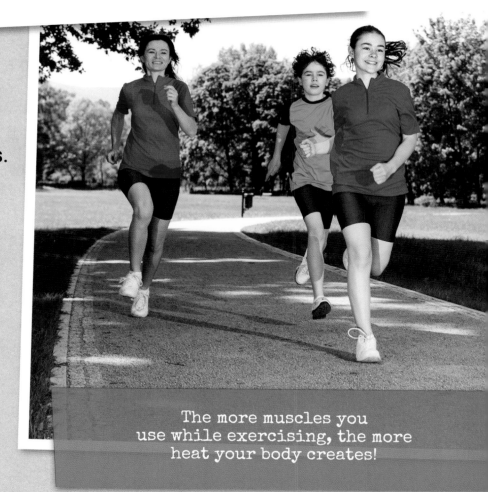

The more muscles you use while exercising, the more heat your body creates!

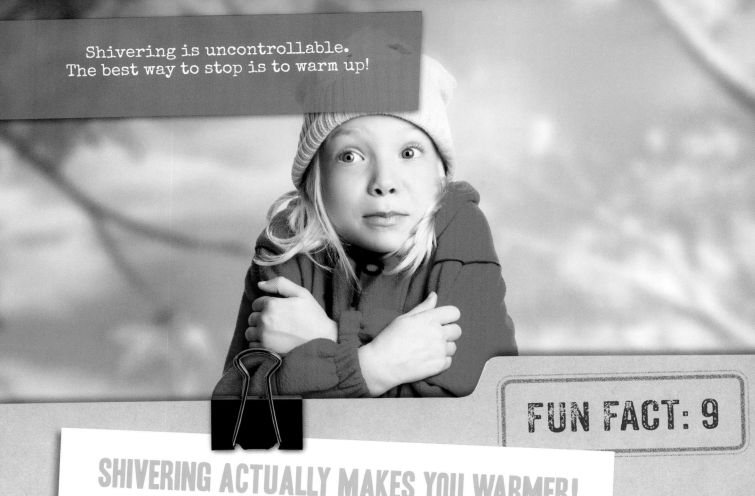

Shivering is uncontrollable.
The best way to stop is to warm up!

SHIVERING ACTUALLY MAKES YOU WARMER!

When you feel cold, your muscles contract and relax very quickly over and over again. This shivering makes heat and warms you up! These muscle movements are involuntary and kick in as soon as your body temperature begins to drop.

ENERGETIC EYES

YOUR EYE MUSCLES ARE THE BUSIEST MUSCLES IN YOUR BODY!

The six muscles attached to each of your eyeballs are constantly moving. This keeps your eyes **focused** while the rest of your body moves. Your eyes can move over 100,000 times a day!

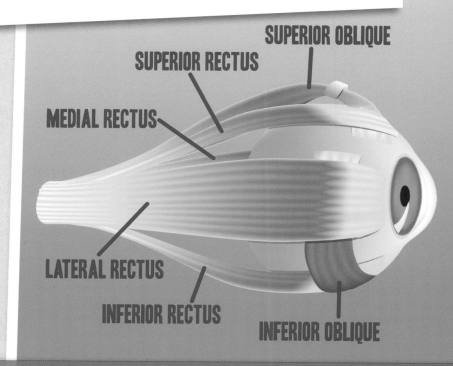

SUPERIOR OBLIQUE

SUPERIOR RECTUS

MEDIAL RECTUS

LATERAL RECTUS

INFERIOR RECTUS

INFERIOR OBLIQUE

Do your eyes ever feel tired? It might be because they can move more than three times per second!

16

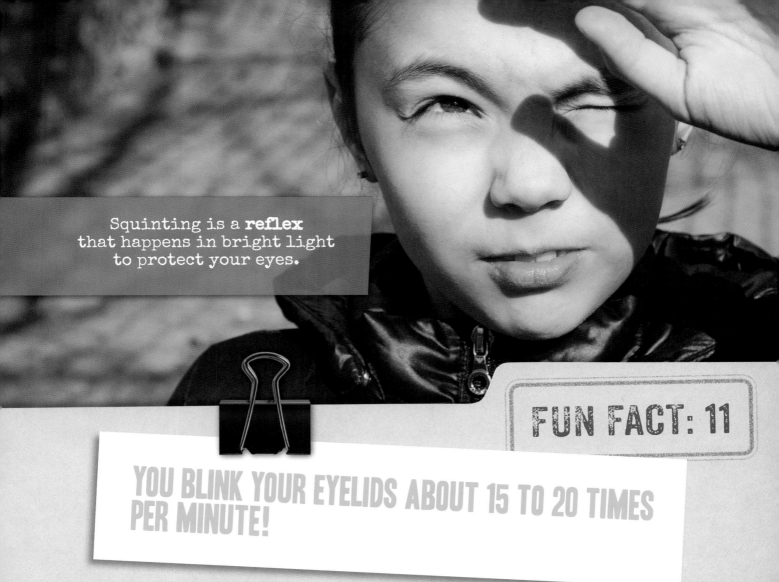

Squinting is a **reflex** that happens in bright light to protect your eyes.

YOU BLINK YOUR EYELIDS ABOUT 15 TO 20 TIMES PER MINUTE!

This keeps your eyeballs from drying out. Blinking is both a voluntary and involuntary muscle movement. You can blink whenever you choose, but sometimes you blink without thinking.

ONE OF THE STRONGEST MUSCLES IN YOUR BODY IS IN YOUR HEAD!

The masseter, or jaw muscle, creates a massive amount of force when it closes. It pulls the lower jaw up to close your mouth. This force helps you to bite and chew your food.

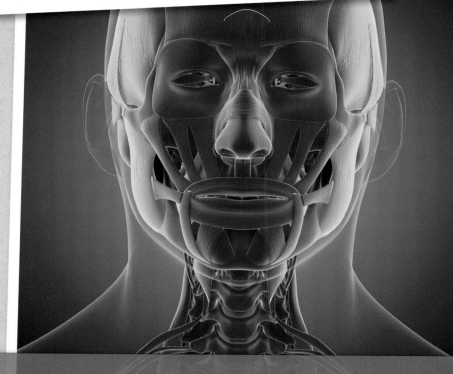

Your jaw muscle is small but powerful!

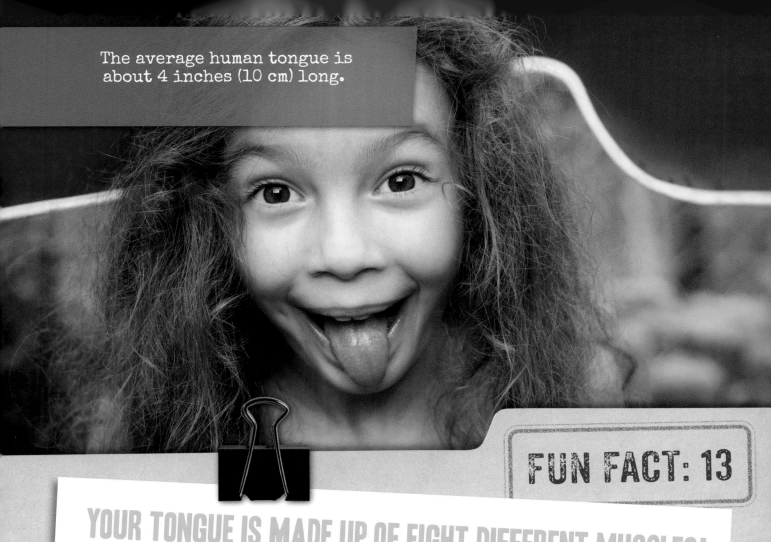

The average human tongue is about 4 inches (10 cm) long.

YOUR TONGUE IS MADE UP OF EIGHT DIFFERENT MUSCLES!

Four muscles in the front of the tongue allow you to change its shape in order to speak. Four muscles in the back move the tongue and connect it to bones in your mouth.

19

THE SMALLEST SKELETAL MUSCLE IS IN YOUR EAR!

The stapedius muscle is less than 0.08 inches (2 mm) long. It's found in the middle ear and **supports** the stapes, which is the smallest bone in your body.

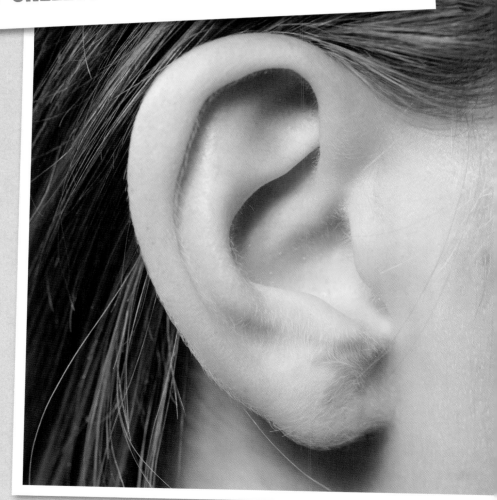

INSIDE THE EAR

STAPES BONE

STAPEDIUS MUSCLE

The stapedius muscle contracts and pulls back the stapes bone. This protects the inner ear from loud sounds.

POWERHOUSE MUSCLES

THE LARGEST MUSCLE IS THE GLUTEUS MAXIMUS.

It's one of three muscles in your bottom that help you keep your balance, climb stairs, and walk uphill. The gluteus maximus, gluteus medius, and gluteus minimus muscles move your thighs in different directions.

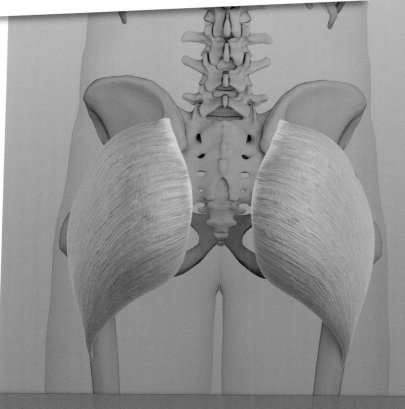

Your gluteus maximus helps you climb stairs and stand up from a sitting position.

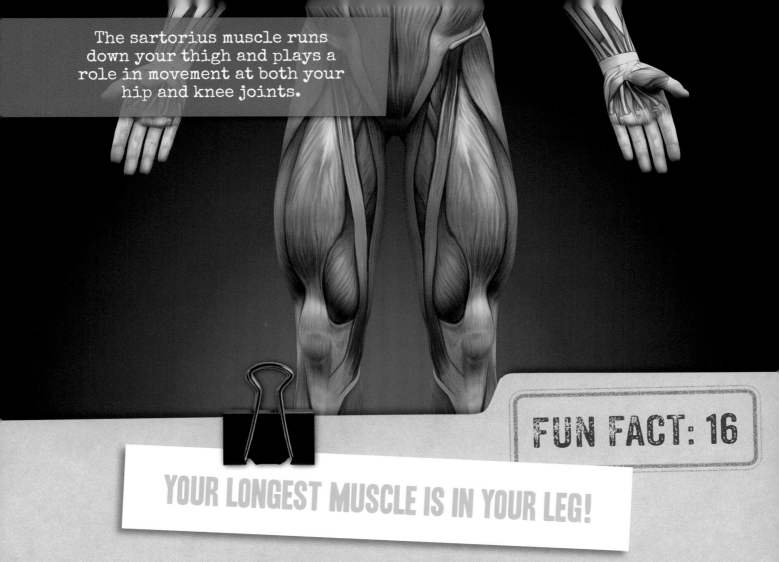

The sartorius muscle runs down your thigh and plays a role in movement at both your hip and knee joints.

YOUR LONGEST MUSCLE IS IN YOUR LEG!

The sartorius muscle connects the front of your pelvis to the upper part of your shinbone. It helps turn your thigh and knee away from your body so you can sit with your legs crossed.

23

STRONG AND SMART

YOUR MUSCLE FIBERS TEAR A TINY BIT WHEN YOU EXERCISE!

When your muscles contract more than they're used to, it causes microtears in the muscle fibers. This can make your muscles feel sore. These tiny tears will make the muscle stronger in the long run.

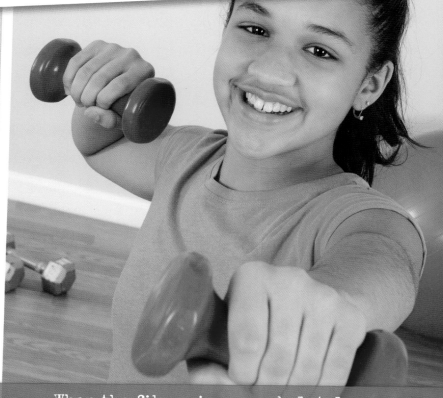

When the fibers in your skeletal muscles tear, more fibers grow to heal the injury. This makes your muscles grow larger and stronger.

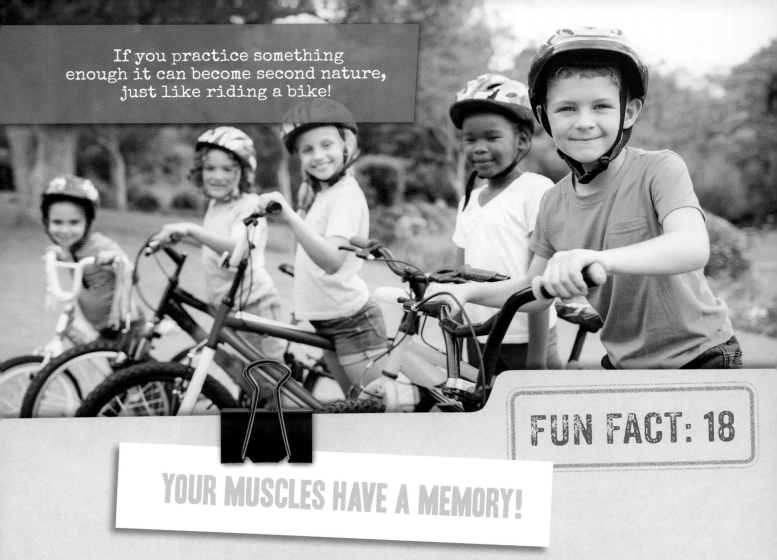

If you practice something enough it can become second nature, just like riding a bike!

YOUR MUSCLES HAVE A MEMORY!

When you repeat a movement again and again, your muscles remember that movement and do it better each time. After a while, your muscles can perform the skill without you thinking about it.

WASTING AWAY

MUSCLES CAN HELP FIGURE OUT WHEN SOMEONE DIED.

A few hours after death, muscle fibers get stuck in a contracted position causing the muscles throughout the body to become stiff. This is called rigor mortis, which is Latin for "stiffness of death." The stages of rigor mortis give clues about someone's time of death.

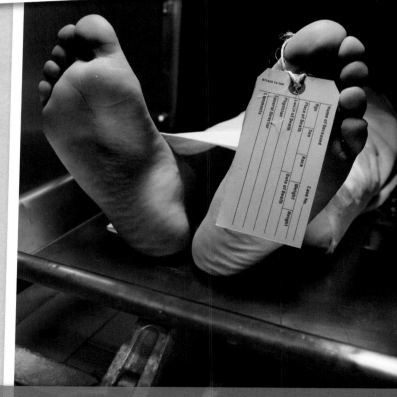

Depending on conditions in the **environment,** the body's muscles will begin to relax again after about 48 hours.

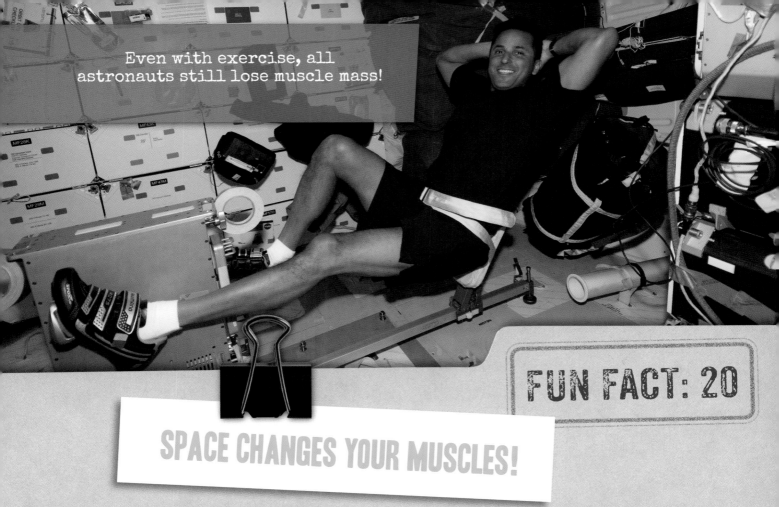

Even with exercise, all astronauts still lose muscle mass!

SPACE CHANGES YOUR MUSCLES!

On Earth, your muscles work against **gravity**. They help you stand upright and pump blood to your heart. In space, these muscles don't have to work as hard, and they begin to waste away. Astronauts have to exercise to keep their muscles healthy!

27

ON THE MOVE

Your muscular system plays an important role in moving your body. Your muscles help you speak, digest your food, and move around. They pump your blood, help you to see, and are even working when you use the bathroom! Some of these muscles need you to tell them what to do, but many work on their own.

In fact, while you have been reading this book, some of your muscles have been hard at work. Can you guess which ones?

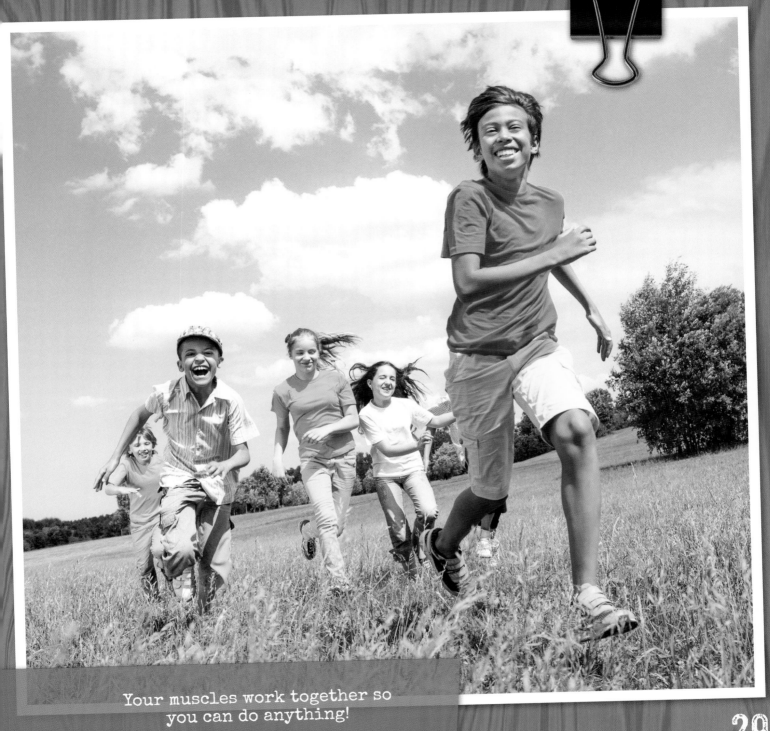

Your muscles work together so you can do anything!

GLOSSARY

cardiac: having to do with the heart

environment: the conditions that surround a living thing and affect the way it lives

fiber: a long, thin piece of material that forms a type of tissue in your body

focus: to adjust to make an image clearer

gravity: the force that pulls objects toward Earth's center

impulse: a small amount of energy that moves from one area to another

intestines: a long tube in the body that helps break down food after it leaves the stomach

joint: a point where two bones meet in the body

nutrient: something a living thing needs to grow and stay alive

organ: a part of the body (such as the heart or liver) that has a certain job

reflex: a reaction to something that you do without thinking

sphincter: a ring-shaped muscle that surrounds a body opening

support: to hold up and help

tendon: a band of tough tissue that connects muscles and bones

vessel: a small tube that carries fluids to different parts of the body

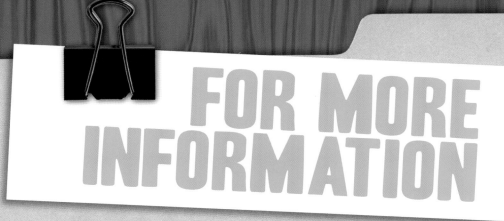

BOOKS

Davies, Kate. *Illumanatomy*. London, England: Wide Eyed Editions, 2017.

Gardner, Jane P. *Take a Closer Look at Your Muscles*. Mankato, MN: The Child's World, 2014.

Mason, Paul. *Your Brilliant Bones and Marvellous Muscular System*. London, England: Hachette Children's Group, 2015.

WEBSITES

Body Systems
www.dkfindout.com/us/human-body/your-amazing-body/body-systems/
Learn more about muscles and other body systems.

Human Biology: The Muscular System
kidsbiology.com/human-biology/muscular-system/
Watch a video about how muscles make the body move.

Your Muscles
kidshealth.org/en/kids/muscles.html
Find fun facts about muscles here.

INDEX